THE ZEN OF BEAUTY

A Guide to Your Magnificence

By Dennis and Jamie Roche

Balboa Press books may be ordered through booksellers or by contacting:

Balboa Press
A Division of Hay House
1663 Liberty Drive
Bloomington, IN 47403
www.balboapress.com
1 (877) 407-4847

ISBN: 978-1-5043-7010-3 (sc)
ISBN: 978-1-5043-7011-0 (e)

Print information available on the last page.

Balboa Press rev. date: 12/16/2016

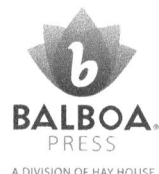

BALBOA
PRESS
A DIVISION OF HAY HOUSE

DEDICATION

We would like to dedicate this book to all those who, at one point in their lives, felt like they were not the best, could not compete or were just not recognized for the potential they owned. You are a special breed, one and all. This is what we will show you within the chapters of this book. Our belief is that you will walk away from this experience with a greater heart and more complete soul.

Special thanks to Michele Orwin for believing in me, Wendi Blum of Flourish Book Club for helping me organize, and my wife Jamie for her grounding forces and boundless encouragement.

And to all the professionals I have had the pleasure of working beside, creating with and learning from.

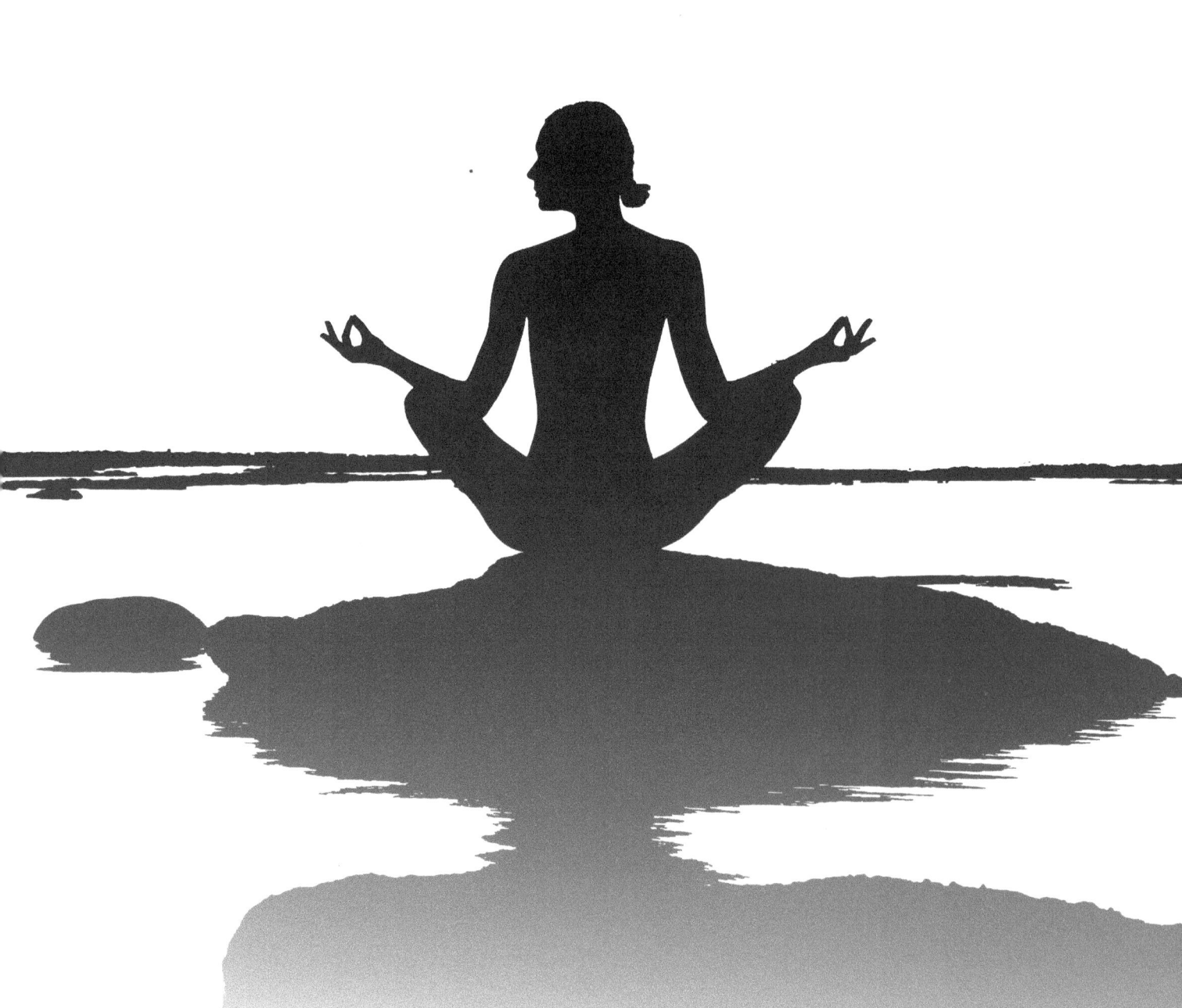

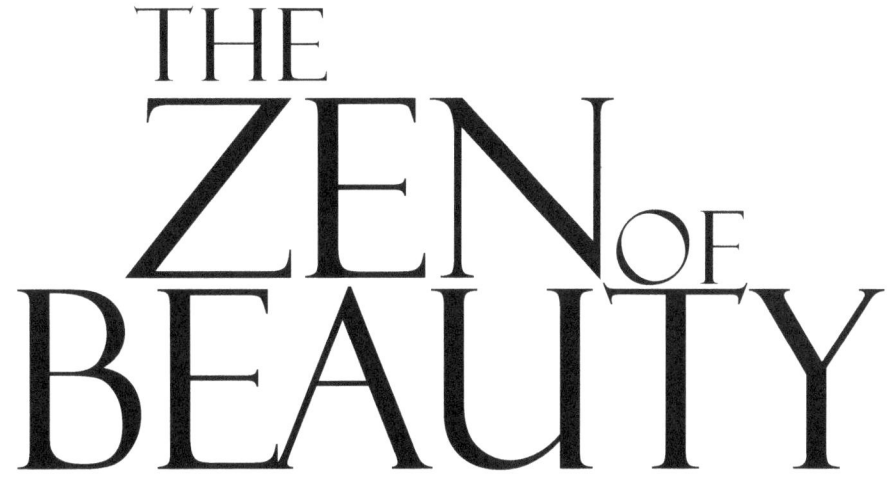

THE ZEN OF BEAUTY

A Guide to Your Magnificence

By Dennis and Jamie Roche

CONTENTS

PREFACE

Today my wife, Jamie, and I embark on one of the greatest adventures of our lives—writing this book. Jamie is a career makeup artist, skin care and retail specialist. I am career hairdresser, salon owner, and beauty expert. *The Zen of Beauty* details our experiences over many years working with clients. Together we wish to share some truths based on our years of experience that will help launch you spiritually and mentally into a newfound inner and outer beauty that will help improve your life.

Throughout our lives we are fed so much information about who we are, that we look like, what we *should* look like—all according to the expectations of others. We are bombarded with images and messages every day that tell us what we are is not good enough. As human beings, we are all unique in our strengths and beauty, how we see ourselves, and how our appearances are perceived by the world. This book is designed to help you take leadership and control of your life, your inner and outer beauty, your overall appearance, and communicate your desires to the army of professionals who will educate you on how to own and create your inner and outer glamour.

Together we will walk down a path toward the light of self-acceptance and bring a real sense of power and peace to the reflection you see in the mirror. Some of what we share in these pages is based on science and others are based on the ultimate belief that you can create a perfect you: strong, sound, confident, and ready to take on the world.

Each chapter includes a meditation and activity to deepen your self-reflection and understanding of the principles discussed. Take your time and complete the activities at the end of each chapter. Be honest and take note of how each exercise can help you in your daily life. You may want to meditate on some of these thoughts, and others you may wish to repeat often to truly understand the process and how this will all serve you best. Take time at the end of each chapter and reflect on the intention of the words. Look in the mirror each morning and repeat your intention and believe that your day will form around it. Present yourself as if your happiness and success were predicated on this intention. Allow yourself to be successful with all that these intentions bring. You will see your existence change and your heart grow with every moment you allow.

Once you finish this book, save it and reread it once in a while and even revisit the exercises to refresh yourself. Being enlightened is a 365, 24/7 full-time job.

Peace & Love
Dennis and Jamie Roche

Chapter 1

GLAMOUR:
THE ILLUSION OF BEAUTY

First, let us explore the difference between glamour and beauty.

If you look back into the history of cinema and fashion and really look closely, not all women famous for their looks were necessarily "beautiful," but reflected a culmination of a group of hair, makeup, and fashion artists who corroborated together with a decisive plan on what they were trying to communicate through the image of that individual.

Some of us are natural at picking out and creating this illusion of glamour through whatever means we learned or innately picked up. I believe those to be few. Most of us stumble through life looking for—but not fully understanding or getting—what we want or desire.

The popular belief is that, "You can't judge a book by its cover." While this is true, you also would not pick a book off the shelf in a bookstore unless that cover gave you a message that there was something important for you to know inside that book. Publishing companies know this, and spend lots of hours and dollars creating a cover that peaks your interest. That is what producers do for upcoming starlets—by forming a goal, creating a team, and changing the image of that person, sometimes even their name, to create the illusion that will make them successful. Marilyn Monroe, Greta Garbo, Joan Crawford, Bette Davis, and most of the iconic women in the last decades all took on a transformation to enhance their image and create the impression that their beauty was something of envy. Many became the style leaders of their eras. The choices were not theirs at first, but the choices made for them to create an illusion that ushered in their fame and success.

You may have read about or heard of some of these women and the tragic personal lives they led. They were not in charge of their own lives. Broken marriages, drugs, alcohol, and suicides were not uncommon among that group of actors, musicians, models, and those living what would seem like dream lives. Their "dream lives" were an illusion. Success was thrown upon them and their public image was not their idea, but that of "owners" and "handlers" wanting to create their own brand of star. They played a role not of their own making, and many paid dearly for not being in control of their image. They were denied the ownership we all need to succeed in bringing out our best. Yes, they were glamorous, but they didn't show their true inner beauty; rather, their beauty was created by others.

Ownership is the key to all your happiness, not just with your appearance, but with your life. *Deciding to decide is an important part of the equation.* It allows you to be free. It allows you to be strong and fearless. It allows you to love yourself and spread that love.

What we are suggesting is that you own your plan, you take the initiative in creating your brand, you take the bull by the horns and give thanks to the universe for your existence and the opportunity to take that perfect you and present it to the world in the manner you choose with the advice that most helps your heart feel true contentment and happiness.

Take ownership of the changes you would like to make in your image—based on what is in your heart. The focus in making changes should be in bringing your inner beauty out for the world to see. We've all been captivated by a person at an event or party, someone who lights up a room and makes you want to meet her. The woman who has her own style, integrated with her life and preferences; she lives with confidence in her uniqueness and individuality, completely comfortable in herself.

We all have that ability. It is a matter of first looking deep inside, being fearless, and allowing ourselves to be successful. As the old adage goes, "There is nothing to fear but fear itself." **Believe** that the effort is worthwhile; the outcome will enable you to feel and see yourself in the greatest light.

To start on your amazing journey requires just that: **believing** and **beginning**!

You are the Universe and it all exists because

you choose it to be. Give thanks to everything, bask in acceptance and feel the gratitude for your life and potential. Focus on the good you have created and let go from your heart all the trespasses you may have felt were part of your decision-making processes.

The only things you risk losing are things that you became comfortable with that actually had no real bearing on your steps forward; virtually remove them from your heart and make room for the real you. This is not an unreal process, just a task like any other you have undertaken in your life. We are all culminations of what has passed, not victims. Think how many times someone told you how perfect you are and how many times words were spoken that hurt your feelings or made you feel inferior. In my professional experience, more clients communicate negative information about themselves from the past and other's opinions, rather than what is pertinent now. Drop those in the trash on your next walk outside; let those things go and let your heart accept your perfection. Those are thoughts for ordinary people and truly enlightened ones hold the truth that they are extraordinary.

You hold the key to all that happens from here on. **Believe**.

There's a moment in the movie *Revenge of the Nerds* when Gilbert stands in front of the entire school and says, "I'm a nerd." Audiences had tears in their eyes. I certainly did, because we all have been at a point where we had to admit to who we truly are, to accept and embrace our authenticity. To be brave enough to admit that we are perfect in ourselves.

In the movie, the crowd starts to slowly come forward and at first his best friends start chanting, "Nerd," then more people come forward and scream louder, "Nerd!" More and more come, all chanting in support. They all know the pain of not being accepted, they all know the hurt of being looked down upon for not fitting into the mold that our society decided upon—a standard most often designed to sell us something. We all have laughed and gawked at the Gilberts in our lives, sneered at them, maybe called them names or in some form tried our hardest to make ourselves feel more powerful by making them feel inferior. It is so much easier to look down on others than be honest to ourselves.

The ones without tears for Gilbert are those who

have become so hardened and jaded; those who gain power for not participating, not caring and not letting their hearts open up to let themselves be vulnerable. Humility is the ability to open your heart enough to see yourself, in all your beauty and perfection. And to see others in the same way.

Meditation:

Sit comfortably and repeat these phrases to yourself: I am whole. I am the perfect me. I am created in the likeness of my God.
Repeat throughout the day.

Activity:

Think of the greatest lesson you have learned from a book, movie, teacher, friend, or life experience about the strength of your authentic personal presentation.

Chapter 2

SYMMETRY AND PERCEPTION

We all have the God-given privilege and blessing of being unique. You are the only *you* that will ever exist in the entire universe. That makes you the perfect you, like no other. Embrace that uniqueness. This is a fact and there is no denying you are a star in this world. If you've had any hesitation or doubt of your worthiness, it is time to drop it right now. No matter what you have been told or who you've been influenced by, those are false realities. Only you are the creator of your reality.

Be blessed by this reality; give thanks and gratitude for this perfection that has been disposed upon you. Once you can adopt this reality, you can do and be anything you wish to be. Yes there are hurdles, yes there are others realities that may be imposed on you and your journey, but once you have absolute belief in your perfection, you become invincible.

Showing the world that individuality becomes a must. Our society has become one that uses fear as a basis of selling us something. Our hair looks awful, we're too fat, too skinny, too short, too tall—oh, and that breath!

Yes, it is important to be self-aware, but it should be to the standards you set for your perfect self in your chosen universe. I realize this may sound contrary to Western beliefs, but what does that matter in terms of your happiness? Just because this season's fashion houses are showing what looks like fifteen-year-old, anorexic models with too little clothing and way too much makeup in provocative poses, this is their reality they are pushing at you—it should have little or no bearing on your perfect universe. This goes for the news, television, radio, and any source of information you're influenced by.

To illustrate my point, there has been a rule of

thumb since the 1950s that there are six shapes of faces: round, oval, square, rectangular, triangular, and heart shaped. This "rule" was thought up by an advertising agency when introducing a makeup line. It is actually ridiculous, considering that there are six billion people in the world. That would mean you have a billion twins out there. Imagine if you had a face like one of these shapes—you would look like a cartoon character.

However, there is the principle of symmetry. Having a symmetrical face is the closest to perfection by fashion standards. Very few people have a perfect symmetry to their face; that is where creating the illusion comes into play. This can be accomplished with makeup and hairstyle. Determining the symmetry of your face is the first step.

Follow this simple exercise and you will see the true shape of your face. Stand in front of a mirror. Take a pencil, chopstick or any thin, straight object and hold it in center of your face, both vertically and horizontally. Now look closely at the balance of your face, left to right and top to bottom. Most faces are slightly rounder or wider on one side than the other. Look at the symmetry of the horizontal and vertical lines of

your face.

Now, with your thumb and forefinger, measure the distance from your hairline to the top of the bridge of your nose, then the distance from the top of the bridge to the bottom of your nose, and again from the bottom of the nose to the end of your chin. Note your measurements on the illustration below.

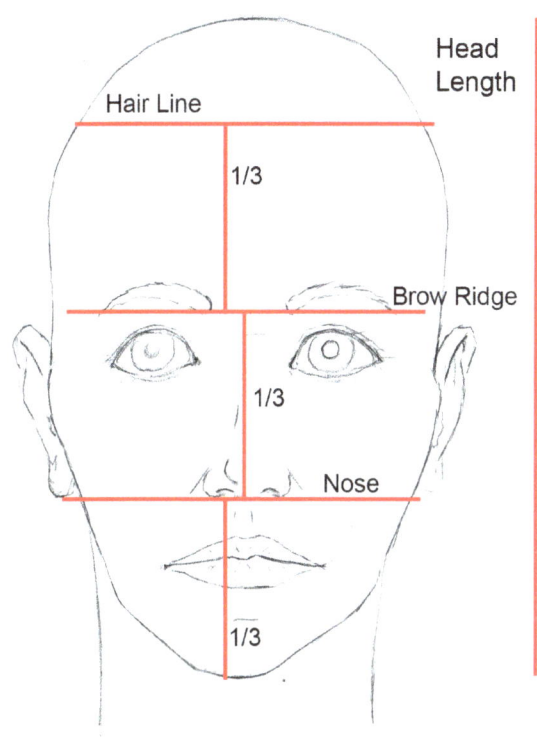

This is the balance and symmetry of your face, pure and simple. No squares, triangles, or weird shapes. This is like a topography map of your face and is essential in helping you choose make

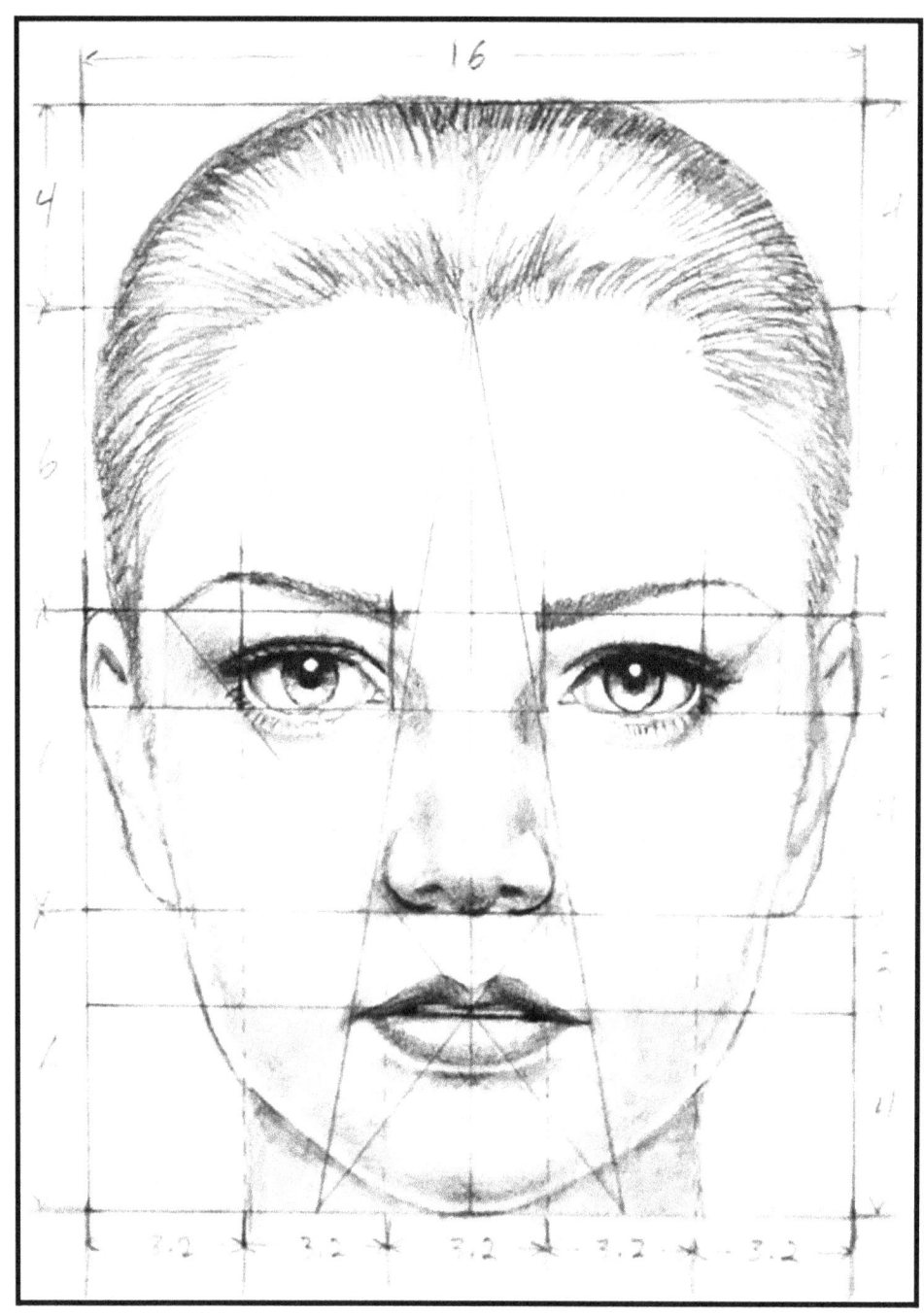

up applications and especially a hairstyle. For example, a short forehead most always means bangs are not the best choice. An asymmetrical haircut should be to the opposite of the narrowest side of your face to create balance. A horizontal imperfection can be visually corrected with a haircut that has opposite asymmetry. Makeup can visually correct lines by extending up or down with an eye pencil, eye shadow, lipstick, blush, or anything that creates horizontal lines on the face.

The human eye only sees what is perceived. This perception can be controlled by altering your makeup or hairstyle. That is where your choices start and where you take control of your projected image.

Arrange your hair and makeup in different ways and take a selfie. Then you can judge for yourself what looks best. And please, don't ask too many people for their opinions. Close friends often do not tell us the truth because of our relationships, and others tell us from their own preferred concepts of acceptability.

This entire chapter is about you and your opinion—and your first step forward to your authentic image. Although "Beauty is in the eye of the beholder," remember that you can create the illusion that will become your message.

Meditation:

Sit comfortably and repeat these phrases to yourself: I am the balance in nature, I am the light of lights, I am the center of the universe. Repeat throughout the day.

Activity:

Using the selfie you like best, draw a picture of your face, taking notice of the dimensions you have measured.

Chapter 3

COLOR ME PERFECT

There are hundreds of lines of colors available in both makeup and hair. How to choose the colors that best suit you can be a considerable challenge and one that baffles most of my clients.

First, let me say that what makes you feel pretty is usually the one that looks best on you.

Choose wisely; have a purpose and goal in mind. Think of your hair color as your background. Is your purpose to blend or contrast, brighten or deepen? In most cases, creating too much of either blending or contrast can be difficult to wear. With too much contrast or lightening, the hair very much demands the use of more make-up to create the proper skin tone. Lightening the background of anything brings out darkness in the foreground. In hair color, it makes imperfections show more dramatically and if you have light eyes, they can lose their brilliance. Darkening the hair too much can create a paleness in the

face that will need additional makeup as well. If you do not like wearing a lot of makeup, then this may not be for you.

Consider the maintenance involved and then monetary and time commitment. Whether going lighter or darker with your hair or makeup, there is a definite need to select the correct tone of color that best compliments your skin tone.

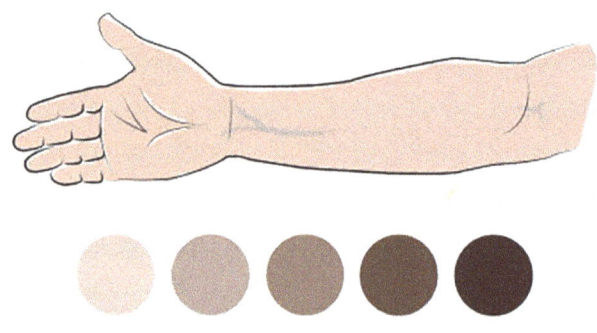

According to the fashion and style industries, there are five basic skin tones according to the books. Again, this puts people in boxes. Skin tones are as unique as we are. Individual skin

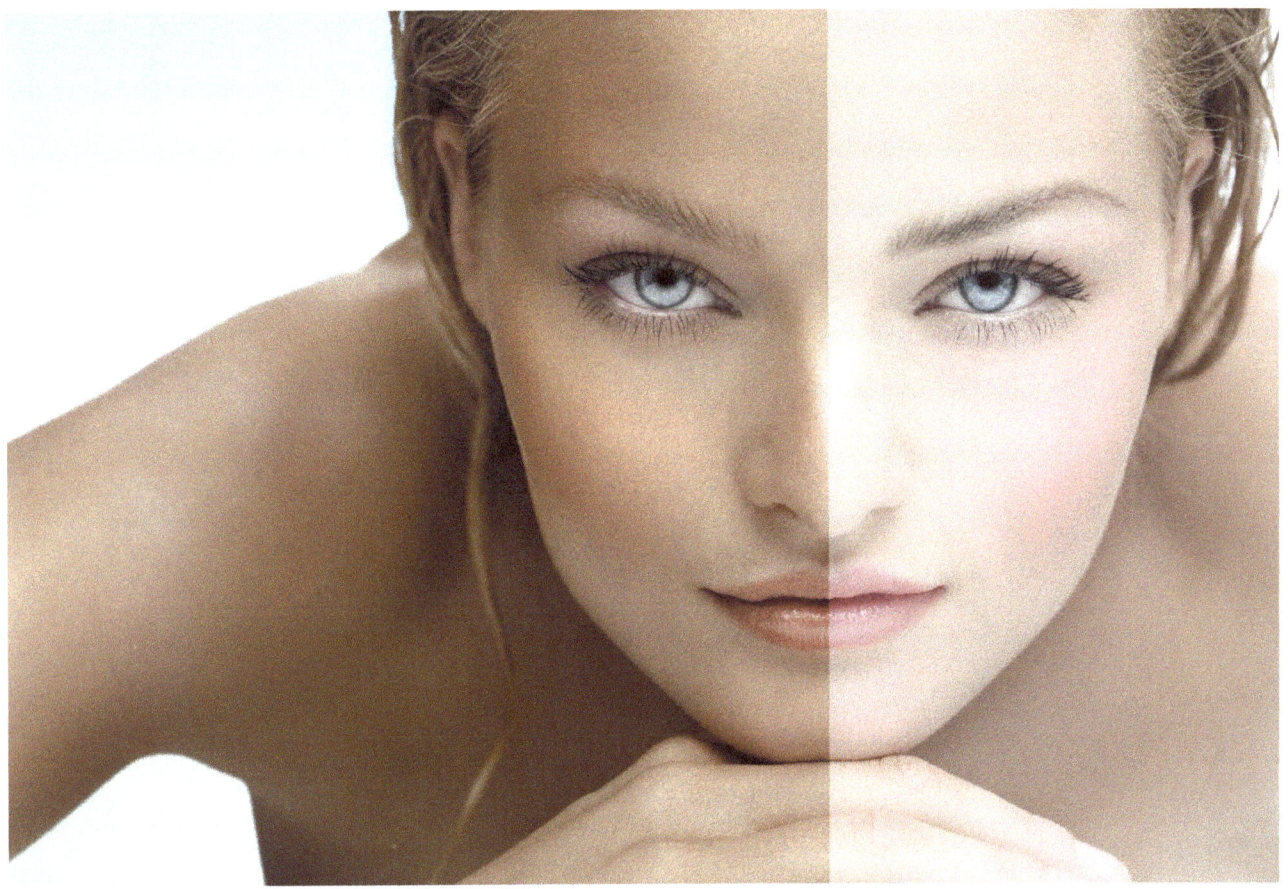

tone is like your fingerprint: it shows up every where but is not generally recognized or at least recognized well by most of us.

When I directed salons at department stores, I would commonly see shoppers, as well as makeup artists, apply colors to the backs of people's hands. Hold the back of your hand against your face, look in a mirror and tell me if there is a similarity. I believe those are skin colors, not tones, and they are not an accurate representation.

Here is the best way of determining your skin tone. The one place with the least amount of tonal changes during your entire life is the inside of your forearm. When checking the tone of any color you wear or are going to use, simply hold it to the inner forearm and observe if it warms or cools your skin tone.

You can do this with color cards or hair swatches to clearly see the color accurately. Whatever the effect of the color is on your inner forearm, it is guaranteed to be the same on your entire body.

"Colors are so important to your life, well-being, and surroundings. In terms of appearances, it shows your character and your personality."

Remember that color changes with light and the eye can be fooled depending on the use of color and light, so for drastic changes or important events, try colors in different lighting before making a final decision. I use this tip for choosing hair color, makeup color, painting a picture, or even painting a wall.

Colors are so important to your life, well-being, and surroundings. In terms of appearances, it shows your character and your personality. I use hair color swatches and hold them against a client's inner forearm. This gives them the chance to see the differences and make an informed decision. Tonal quality is like describing the sense of smell; it is vague unless compared to something else. As important as it is, it gets overlooked by most of us and guessing can be frustrating. Leaving it up to someone else is relinquishing ownership. Understanding this principle and checking colors against your own skin tone is invaluable.

Using this simple tool, I cannot tell you the amazing results clients have in choosing hair color, makeup, clothing and accessories and the confidence they show in taking ownership when doing so.

Mediation:

Sit comfortably and repeat these phrases to yourself: I close my eyes and let my mind go. I see the colors of my heart. Let them shine and take me to my glory.
Repeat throughout the day.

Activity:

Take some different colored cloths and hold them to your inner forearm. Notice the tonal change of your skin and the effect. The same effect will happen to your face tone when you surround it with that color. Repeat the exercise with different colors. Write down the three colors that work best.

1._____

2._____

3._____

Chapter 4

CLEANING HOUSE

Studies have estimated that the average woman owns just shy of forty makeup products and fifteen hair care products. Considering that mascara and eyeliner and anything you use near your eyes has a shelf life of about three to four months once opened, it's probably time to go through your makeup drawer and clean house. Hair care products have a longer life, but remember they are organic and their effectiveness still diminishes over time.

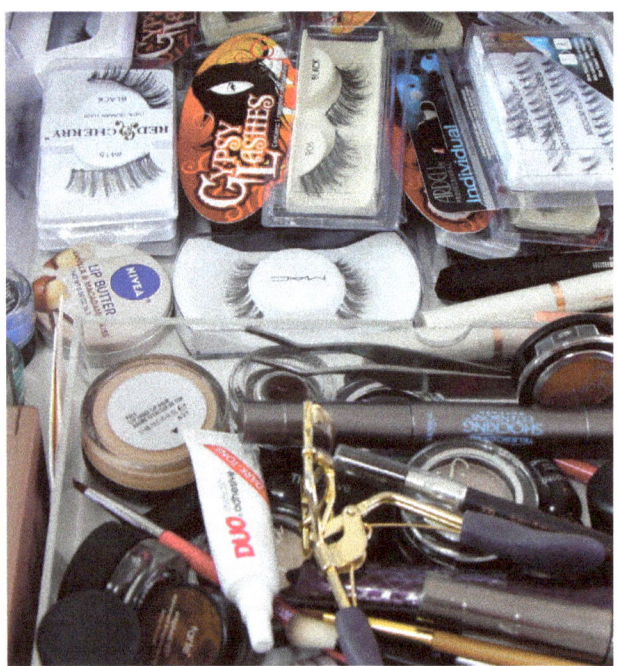

Also, most women were taught about applying makeup when they were teens—and that is usually the last training they had. Now, considering your age, your position in life, and your career success, it may be time to reevaluate the current way you are doing your makeup.

The same goes for your hair. Nothing makes you look older than looking dated. You owe it to yourself and to your spouse, lover, coworkers, and anyone else you are in constant contact with to update yourself. This is a must, particularly in your professional life. Your significant other will so appreciate the new woman you are becoming, and your confidence bell will ring off the hook. It's possible that even your love life will flourish!

On the job and in the workplace, you will gain a newfound respect from coworkers and superiors. Consider two people doing the exact same job with the same level of performance. Who will

"Considering that mascara

and eyeliner and anything

you use near your eyes has a shelf life of

about three to four months once opened,

it's

probably time to go through your makeup

drawer and

clean house."

the boss give the promotion to: the old gal over there, steadfast but true, or the competent woman whose appearance would best represent the business and look the part of management? Who would you pick?

It's an old axiom that change is the only constant in life. As a makeup artist and hairdresser for forty-plus years, constant training and participation in shows was key to staying contemporary and popular with clients and agencies. This took a considerable amount of time, planning, and diligence to stay current with trends in the industry, but without it I wouldn't have the success I have had. This culminates in what and how to advise and please our clients, and we have seen proven success.

Within these chapters are the shortcuts you can use to determine exactly what you want your image to communicate to the world, and to also be able to communicate your desires to your trusted hair stylists and makeup artists. You now know where you want to go, and you can make these changes at whatever pace works for you.

Ask yourself, and be honest in your answer: "Is my current image what I would like to show the world? Do I reflect the contemporary styles with grace and ease? Do I project my position with my presence?"

The way forward is to know exactly what you want and what works best for you, which can be contemporary or timeless, but not dated. And to reproduce it on a regular basis, you must know exactly what you want and have the team of your chosen professionals be clear on your innermost wishes.

Meditation:

Sit comfortably and repeat these phrases to yourself: I am a unique star in the universe. I will show those around me my inner beauty with my personally designed outer beauty. Repeat throughout the day.

Activity:

Write three sentences about your intentions with the improvements you wish to make in your image.

1._____

2._____

3._____

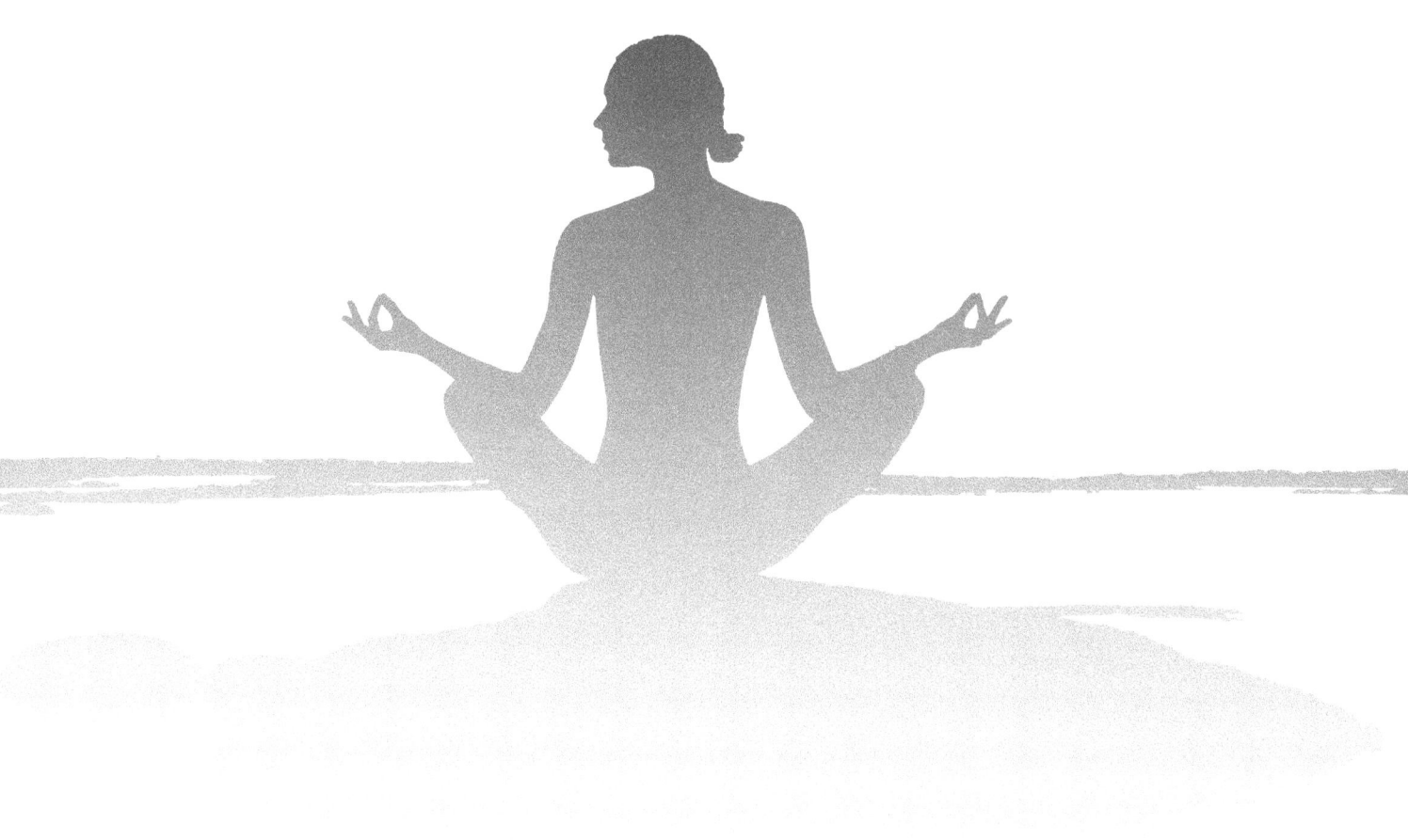

Sit comfortably and repeat these phrases to yourself:

I am a unique star in the universe. I will show

those around me my inner beauty with my person-

ally designed outer beauty.

Repeat throughout the day.

"This is the most harrowing chapter of all! In my forty-year career, I can remember on one hand the clients who told me they liked their hair textures. Typically women complain that their hair is too thin, too thick, too wavy, too curly, or too straight. The bottom line is that they are unhappy with their hair."

Chapter 5

HAIR TEXTURES

This is the most harrowing chapter of all! In my forty-year career, I can remember on one hand the clients who told me they liked their hair textures. Typically women complain that their hair is too thin, too thick, too wavy, too curly, or too straight. The bottom line is that they are unhappy with their hair.

Technology today has made great strides in hair care products, straighteners, and even temporary waves. As a practical matter, it makes sense to use your natural texture, but sometimes the texture is just too wild or stringy or flat. Haircuts and proper training from your hairdresser can make up for any lack in texture. A very important part of the process is to make choices based on your comfort level, needs, budget, and time you want to spend on your hair. Also, take into consideration that you are on the precipice of a new image—your horizons are broadening.

This a clear case of needing good professional help. A skilled hairdresser with proper training can really help you at this stage. Not all hairdressers are as good with some textures as others. Ask lots of questions. When requesting an appointment, ask for the stylist who is the best with hair texture like yours—the receptionist always has a handle on who does what best. Always have a consultation with your stylist first and be open and frank about your challenges in styling your hair. Do not be afraid to speak your mind or even interview several stylists before having services done.

In addition, the next time you book an appointment with your hair stylist, ask for an extra fifteen minutes to have the stylist thoroughly show you how to achieve your desired style. While you are at it, have him suggest the proper products within your budget to be able to finish the style, and their proper use. Do not be afraid to invest in the products, as they will save you so much time and effort. Professional products are exactly that—they are better!

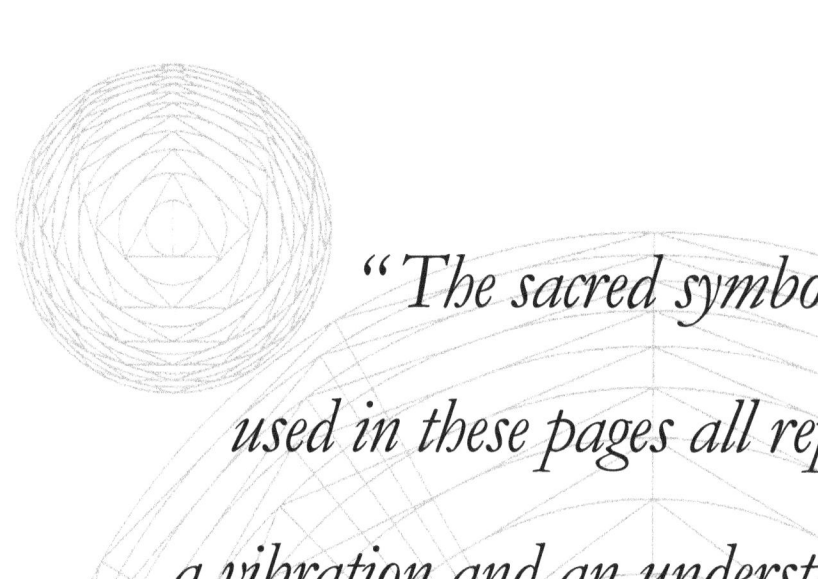

"*The sacred symbols*

used in these pages all represent

a vibration and an understanding in

our life.

Just like our hair, we can choose to

recognize and accept them or alter or

change them.

The choice is always yours

and yours alone."

Hydrolyzed proteins absorb into the hair better and protect the moisture balance and manageability. I recommend you use the shampoo advised by your stylist. The real trick to conditioning your hair well is to put a quarter-sized dollop in the palm of your hand, dab a comb into the conditioner, and comb a small amount from the ears down until it is nearly all gone. What small amount of conditioner is left in the palm should be applied to the top of the head and combed through. Rinse the top of your head, but do not thoroughly rinse the ends.

Like any moisture, moisture in hair evaporates. The more that remains in the ends, the longer your hair will stay at its best texture. Remember, all professional products contain sunscreen. In fact, I recommend that clients mix a small amount of sunscreen to their hair in sunny, hot climates to help protect their investment. This is especially true for redheads and blondes, because those colors tend to fade the fastest.

Brushing your hair thoroughly several times a day prevents you from needing to wash it as much. Washing your hair, especially long hair and color-treated long hair, is singularly the harshest thing you can do to your hair. Do the math: washing your hair every day means 365 times a year; every other day is 182 times a year; and every three days is 122 times a year. When you add blow-drying, ironing, curling, or even naturally drying, this is a lot of wear and tear on your hair.

Meditation:

Sit comfortably and repeat this phrase to yourself: I have been blessed with the potential to have all the goodness in my heart show in my glamour.
Repeat throughout the day.

Activity:

List three things about your daily beauty regimen and how you can improve on it.

1._____

2._____

3._____

Chapter 6

LOSING IT IN TRANSLATION

How many times have you or your friends complained that the stylist working with you did not listen to what you said or wanted? How many times was your vision not anything like the outcome? How many times have you asked the stylist what to do with your hair, rather than owning your own choices?

As a hair professional for more than forty years, I would have to say consistency is the single hardest thing for a hair stylist. So much depends on the education and the diligence of any particular stylist. The best ones keep abreast of technologies and trends by attending a lot of trainings. In my case, I pursued companies I could work for during trainings and stage work and have had the advantage of hundreds of thousands of dollars worth of education. Jamie and I also work on fashion shows, art fashion shows, and photography shoots to keep our creative juices flowing. Unfortunately, that is the exception in my industry.

Part of my hope for this book is not only to encourage women to upgrade their image and make their own choices about what image they want to project, but also to inform professionals on how to consult with clients clearly and obtain the most satisfying results.

First, you must be willing to relinquish the past and take the culmination of knowledge gained from this book and move it into the future. Like makeup and hair products, they all have a shelf life and, like old thoughts and beliefs, need to be either discarded or updated to create a new you. **Your willingness is your success**.

There is a way to check my theory. Pull out some old pictures of yourself and then take a selfie and look at the progression of your image over the years. Would you hire or promote the person you see? Is there room for improvement? For most women, the questions usually become: "Where do I start and who in the world is going to help me design this? Where will I find these people on my budget and is it necessary to throw out everything and start over?"

These are the questions we need to ask ourselves. Getting started and into the process is not as hard as you might think. In fact, with a little effort and following the prescribed outlines in this book, women on any budget and within any time constraints can create the path to personal perfection. Whatever that is for you.

We all laugh at our old pictures and wonder how we could we have loved that perm so much? OMG! That outfit we loved is so silly looking now. The shoes, accessories, hair, and makeup all look dated now, and nothing makes you look older than being dated.

Finding a contemporary solution is within your grasp and achievable if you have a plan. This is where we start having fun and letting our creativity work for us. It is not about being trendy or outrageous, but about being tastefully different and letting our good senses and taste lead us in a new direction.

Meditation:

Sit comfortably and repeat these phrases to yourself: I am free to believe in my inner and outer beauty. I am free from comment and criticism. I am free to open my heart and let the truth of who I am show through.
Repeat throughout the day.

Activity:

Paste a picture here that represents your favorite recent look. Write three words that best describe it.

1._____

2._____

3._____

Chapter 7

THE PATH

When working with clients for the first time, Jamie and I both look with a noncritical eye at a person and try to get a feel for who they are. We notice their purse, shoes, and jewelry and try to determine more about them personally. On Saturdays is the hardest time to do this, because people usually come in on Saturdays very casually dressed, and it is hard to tell a person's style when they're wearing shorts and tennis shoes.

We ask pertinent questions about a client's lifestyle, job, and commitment to their hair and makeup. Are they very low maintenance, or do they mind spending the time to achieve the look they want? Often they ask for my advice on the latest style. My reply is to always ask, "What is your favorite fashion magazine?"

My belief is that you tend to read what you like best. If your inclination is *Vogue,* then that is the type of style you like. *Glamour, Harper's Bazaar* and all the rest feature different looks and styles and their own take on new trends. Each magazine has its own style, which is often reflected by its advertisers.

Most clients use language to communicate their desires, but there is a danger in using words, which is why I ask about favorite fashion magazines. Most of us do not always say what we mean, and this leaves the expert doing what they think best, which may not be exactly what you are saying. This is where all the danger lies.

So it's time to bring out the magazines. We always have an ample supply in the salon, and we go through a few with clients and they tell us what they like or are most inclined to move toward. Of course, this is a lengthy process and I have to add additional time to go through it with clients. It is incredibly successful, but can get expensive for clients. It also can take clients by surprise and put them on the spot to answer questions for which they are unprepared and have had little time to consider.

This is when we came up with the idea of creating a path for clients to be able to bring their own visual to the consultation, which would concisely communicate what they liked, without leaving it up to our translation of their words.

When preparing for a fashion show, advanced education, filming, stage, photo shoots, fashion shows, and even concerts, we create what is known as a "storyboard." This is a map of exactly what the production will look like and the feelings it will generate. The storyboard ensures that everyone involved in the production is on the same page and aligned to keep the focus on the desired effect and what needs to be done.

This is where the "Book of Me" comes into play. There will be a number of experts involved in your personal creation: hairdressers, makeup artists, wardrobe stylists, and jewelers. How do you get them all to have a personal understanding of exactly what you desire? No matter how well we try to communicate to professionals what we want,

and the changes we're looking to make, it always comes down to the interpretation of others.

Meditation

Close your eyes and take three slow, deep breaths. Repeat this line twenty times.

" I allow myself to picture the perfect me, I allow myself to see the images of a perfect life."

Activity:

Write down three descriptive words you would tell your stylists that you believe will describe where you are headed.

1._____

2._____

3._____

Now look up these words in the dictionary and see what the exact definition of the words are in comparison to what you were trying to communicate.

Chapter 8

THE "BOOK OF ME"

To arrive at any desired destination, you have to have a road map. I know today we operate with GPS most of the time, but bear with me when I say a map. As any educator will advise you, write down your plans or goals and they will almost always happen. This works with daily chores, weekly events, special occasions, goals, life dreams, or just about anything you can think of.

If you make writing down your plans or goals an essential part of your daily activities, you will soon make your time and intentions much more effective. In application to our concept of improving or changing your visual perception, writing down what you want becomes everything.

A visual means of presenting our intentions is invaluable. It also narrows our focus and makes us communicate more concisely and clearly. Think of a vision board; when we put our greatest desires in visual form, something magical happens and there's a much greater probability of achieving those desires.

To create your "Book of Me," you'll need your favorite fashion magazines, a piece of paper as large as you wish but big enough to get on it all the information you want (or you can use the blank pages in this book and keep all the information together for updates), and glue. I recommend an 8 x 10-inch poster board, Elmer's glue, an open mind, and a little creativity.

Do not be intimidated; you want to be free with the pictures. The ultimate goal is for you to be able to relate your desires and feelings to your hair stylist and makeup artist to allow them to get an absolutely clear vision of where you want to go with this creation. Page slowly through the magazines and cut out all the pictures you see of things you like. These pictures should be of things that especially pertain to your taste, lifestyle, habits, and professional life.

Are you active in sports, does your job include a great deal of travel, are you active after work and need that quick change from work to play? All these things are what your experts need to know and in as short a time and as accurately as possible.

Every well-intended and well-trained professional takes great pride in their knowledge and service to their clients. Nothing is as daunting as that first experience with a client and trying to not only decipher their desires and needs in such a short period of time, but also delivering the outcome they expect. Stylists will think you are brilliant to have all this to present in such a precise and creative way.

You will give them inspiration, and as an artist there is nothing better than inspiration. You will also get what you pay for. This "Book of Me" will serve as a reminder the next time you see your stylists. A busy hair stylist has eight to ten clients each day, five days a week. And it's often five to six weeks until you return, so this reminder is very important.

Again, this is my consistency theory and how hard it is for professionals to stay on track and current with all of their clients. Part of being a good hairdresser is being a good record keeper, but on a crunched day when clients run late, remembering from five weeks previously what a client's goal is can be a tall task. It's much easier for you to stay on track with yourself and remind your stylists when you see them. We have worked with some of our clients for twenty or thirty years, so I know this works. Haircuts always have a slight difference from appointment to appointment, and hair color always needs tweaking depending on the time of year and the weather. So clear communication with your stylists each time is of the greatest importance.

This book becomes your guideline to update as you like. It will always be there to show your makeup artist or the clerk in you favorite boutique. It gives you complete control in the outcome without the stress, guessing, or bother that comes with returning merchandise or getting a hairstyle you don't like.

Reflect on the lessons given in this book. You will own your own image, it will be everything you desire, and all you have to offer will be recognized by the world. You will walk in beauty, glamour, and most important—confidence.

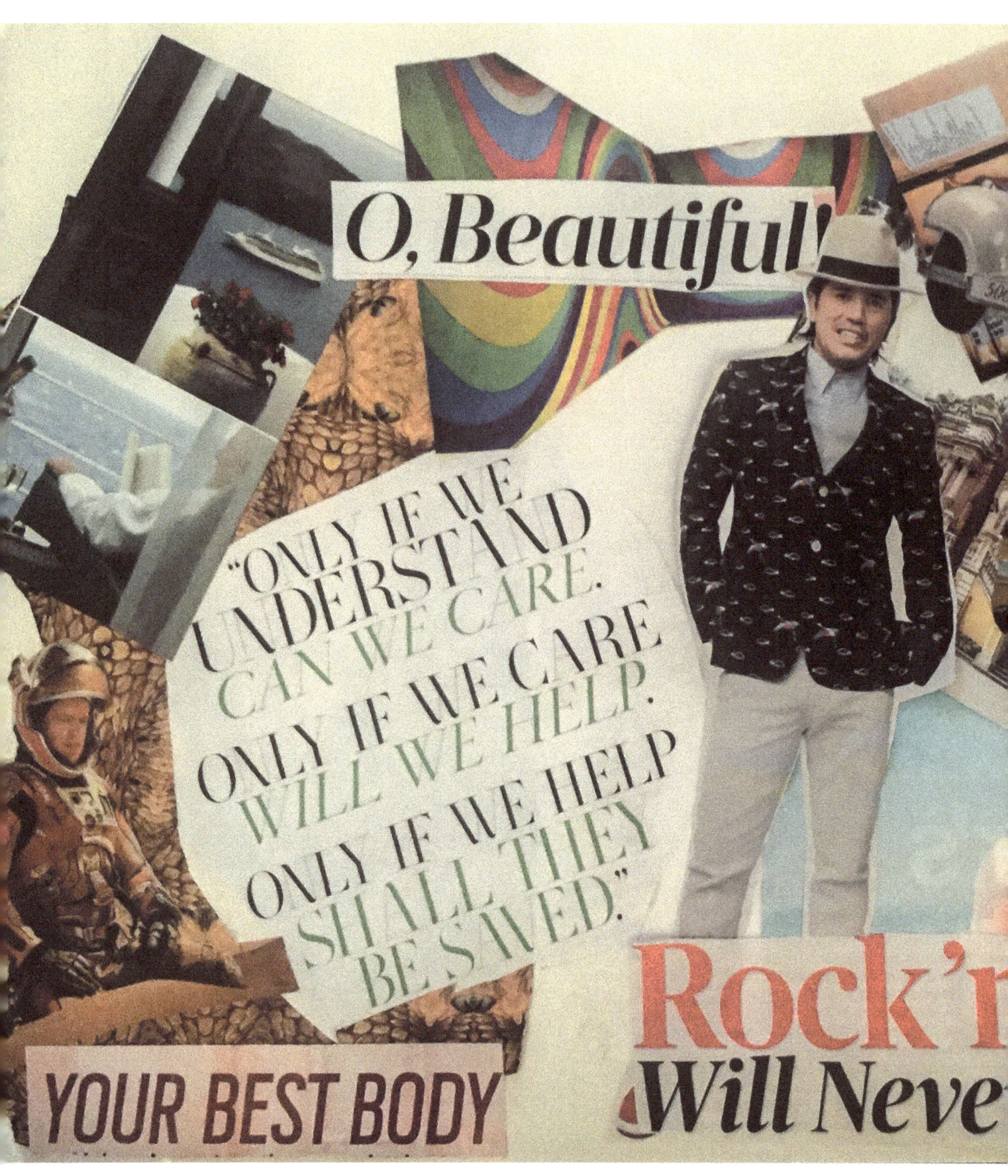

O, Beautiful!

"ONLY IF WE UNDERSTAND CAN WE CARE. ONLY IF WE CARE WILL WE HELP. ONLY IF WE HELP SHALL THEY BE SAVED."

YOUR BEST BODY

Rock'r
Will Neve

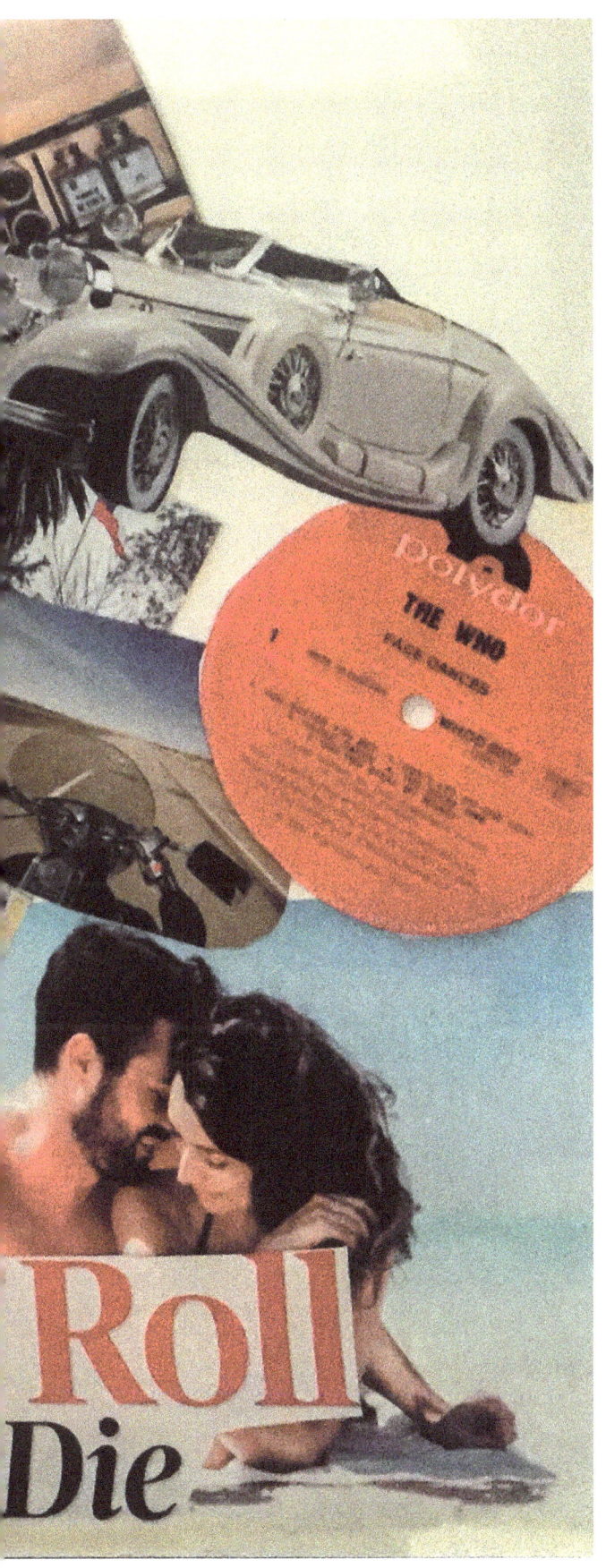

Meditation:

Sit comfortably and repeat these phrases to yourself: I believe that I can have all I want from this world. I believe that I have all that I need to succeed. I feel empowered to release from my heart all negative feelings and love myself.

Repeat throughout the day.

Activity:

Cut out twelve pictures that express your feelings about your beauty. These can include makeup, hairstyles, fashion, or anything else. Arrange them on the following blank pages in the order of your choice. This collage will be your expression and feelings about how you would like to be perceived by your family, friends, and associates. Keep this with you every time you shop or go to a salon or makeup artist. You will have created from within your heart a confidence that will make your shining star brighter.

YOUR "BOOK OF ME" HERE

YOUR "BOOK OF ME" HERE

Chapter 9

TEN BEST HAIR
AND MAKEUP TIPS

"Dennis' Best Hair Tips"

1. If you are an active person or work out a lot, just rinsing your hair and adding conditioner is better than washing. Perspiration is salt water. Rinsing removes it and there is no fatty tissue on your scalp to cause fermentation or, in other words, a bad odor.

2. Brushing your hair several times daily promotes healthier hair. Hair follicles feed on blood circulation alone. Brushing your hair distributes natural oils, relieves you of constant over-washing, and leads to healthier hair.

3. Use a proper brush. Natural bristles are great, but require constant sanitizing. Bacteria and germs constantly build up in them. I recommend a mix of nylon and natural bristles because they require less maintenance and result in less static.

4. Look for conditioners that contain color. They help prevent fading, especially on blonde and red hair, which tend to fade quickly. Ask your stylist's advice on which is best for you.

5. Never use a hot tool that is over 375 degrees. That is scientifically the perfect temperature for any hair styling tool, but above that is damaging.

6. Ask your stylist for protective sprays to use, along with hot tools that best help hold and protect your hair. Do not overuse hot tools. Anything in life you do to an extreme is usually not good for you.

7. Always invest in the best products for your hair. You and your hair are worth it. Use them wisely. Professional products are very concentrated and require a lot less to be effective. The most complaints I have ever heard about professional hair care products were from people who overused them.

8. Keep a comb in your shower to apply conditioner properly. Dabbing conditioner from your hand onto a comb, and beginning from the top

Brushing your hair several times daily promotes healthier hair. Hair follicles feed on blood circulation alone. Brushing your hair distributes natural oils, relieves you of constant over-washing, and leads to healthier hair.

of the ears down, evenly distributes less product more effectively. What is left on your hand can be distributed through the top of your head. Rinse the top of the head more thoroughly and leave most of the product in the ends.

9. Do not overuse products. It is a waste of money and makes the job of styling your hair harder. Over-conditioning or using too much conditioner can make drying your hair harder. It will lead to flat hair that gets dirty faster.

10. Cutting your hair a little more often makes sense. If you want grow out your hair, remember that it only grows one-half inch a month. But it will break more than a half inch if you wait too long for a cut. The rule of thumb when growing out your hair is to trim it every ten to twelve weeks. If you want to maintain the same style, get a cut every six to eight weeks, depending on the style. Waiting longer will result in an overgrown style and you will not get the desired effect.

Jamie's Best Makeup Tips

1. Primer is applied to every canvas before painting. Using a foundation primer appropriate for dry , oily or normal skin is essential, even if you do not use foundation. The benefit is a smoother, healthier skin appearance.

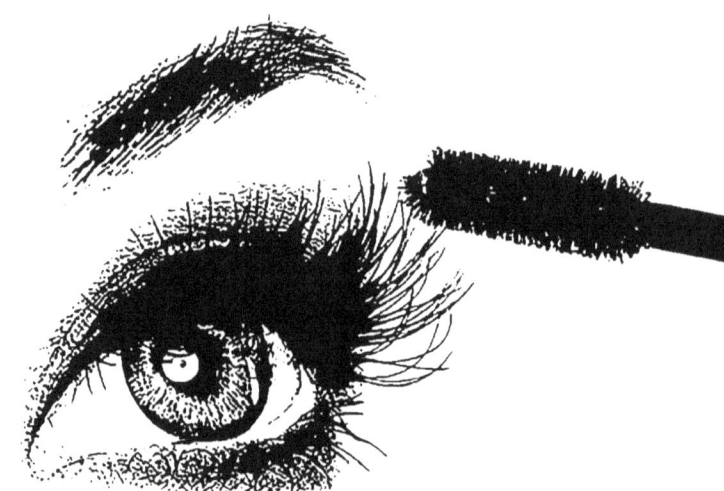

2. Curl your eyelashes and then apply mascara. This is another basic must, no matter how much makeup you wish to use.

3. Use a primer base specific to the eye and then apply over the entire eyelid. Shadow and liner become much easier to use and are longer lasting. Resting your elbow against a counter or wall is helpful to steady your application.

4. A quality brush will give you the best result with a translucent powder. It will set the foundation and give you the absolutely best, smoothest finish. For adverse weather—or to be photographed—use a dual purpose mattifying and hydrating powder.

5. Use creme blushes for a subtle bit of color on the apple of the cheek, followed by a bit of powder blush. This gives a long lasting, natural color to the complexion.

6. If you use a bronzer, remember that less is more and use a very light hand, gently stroking in a W pattern.

7. Always finish under the chin and neck with a little bronzer.

8. For lips, lipsticks, glosses, stains, and crayons are available. Check color tones as explained earlier, on the inside of your forearm. The color you use should compliment the color of your clothes. Own a small collection: soft and sheer for the day, and richer and deeper for the evening. Color glosses can be used on top to change the tone and are also good for using up those mistake purchases.

9. Concealers go on last. Add a tiny drop of serum or eye cream to a concealer; it makes it go on easier and is better for control. For dark circles, use a peach shade of concealer.

10. Your entire collection of neutral tones can be transformed by the choice of lip color, even when going from daytime to night.

ABOUT THE AUTHOR

Dennis Roche (Washington, DC) is a salon owner, mentor, international educator, and author featured in Vogue, Harper's Bazaar, Self, Glamour, and Vanity Fair.

Jamie Roche is a makeup artist, retail expert, and educator for Bobby Brown, Channel, Tom Ford, and Kevin Aucoin.

Together, they bring thousands of client experiences in their beauty guide.

www.ingramcontent.com/pod-product-compliance
Lightning Source LLC
Chambersburg PA
CBHW041131280526
45792CB00013B/2384